P.S., from God

Amy Hillenburg

PUBLISHED BY FIDELI PUBLISHING, INC.

© Copyright 2017, Amy Hillenburg

All Rights Reserved.

No part of this book may be reproduced, stored in a retrieval system, or transmitted by any means, electronic, mechanical, photocopying, recording, or otherwise, without written permission from the author.

ISBN: 978-1-60414-957-9

For information, please contact

Fideli Publishing, Inc.:
info@fidelipublishing.com

www.FideliPublishing.com

This book is dedicated to all those who are still suffering from some form of leukemia, and/or receiving treatments, as well as to those who have lost their lives fighting it. The hope is that more research and additional bone marrow donors will allow longer lives and possibly a cure for this devastating disease.

P.S.,
from God

Table of Contents

Prelude 9

CHAPTER 1
A Dream Interrupted 11

CHAPTER 2
A Nun with a Purpose 27

CHAPTER 3
My Story: How I came to know Christ 41

CHAPTER 4
A Dog from My Mother 45

CHAPTER 5
A Hot-Air Celebration 59

About the Author? 70

Prelude

I wrote this book because there are many people who believe in God, but they think he is only concerned with the overall big picture. He loves us, but he doesn't have time to micromanage our lives. He only gives us direction.

I claimed Jesus Christ in the Methodist Church at age 10. I've always attended church and I've always loved God.

My father was a deacon, and my mom taught Sunday school. But it wasn't until my husband was saved and suddenly fell ill with acute leukemia that I learned we serve a God who's in the details. He cares for each of us individually and gives us exactly what we need when we need it.

God is never an absentee landlord.

His approach is subtle, but you always know the gift is from Him. My journey of true faith started when I became uncomfortable in my old church and joined a new one. It was filled with men who befriended my husband and believed that eventually, Jerry would become a Christian.

When one of these men had a bout with back trouble, a ticket became available to Promise Keepers. It had my husband's name on it, P.S., from God. Another church member led Jerry down the aisle to claim Christ.

He returned that night, hugging me with tears in his eyes.

"I feel like a new person," he said. Indeed, he was.

CHAPTER 1

A Dream Interrupted

My husband Jerry and I were on the brink of a wonderful new start. He had just retired at age 50 from a 35-year career in custom cabinetry and woodworking. He ran his own business, hired his own employees and made sure they had work all year long.

Running your own business is not easy, and you are never really away from it. I was relieved when Jerry decided to take another route to earning an income.

He had worked for mainly one or two builders, and his family members all ran their own shows. His brother Don was a framer, his brother Gary was a home builder, his father Willard began the building business and also sold real estate, his brother Steve was an interior designer. Only his brother Ernie worked for someone else. Yet, he was well versed in homebuilding and woodworking. His adopted brother Mike also runs a painting business.

The year was 2002, and the country was still reeling over the tragic deaths of Sept. 11, 2001 — or 9/11 as we came to call the horrendous day of terrorist attacks on our own soil.

We lived in a small house among the trees in Waverly Woods about 12 miles north of Martinsville, the Morgan County seat. Jerry and his brothers and cousins helped build the two-bedroom home for us before we were married July 15, 1972. Our boys were born there and both graduated from Mooresville High School.

One son was already married. So to prepare for impending grandchildren, we wanted a bigger place. Jerry developed a wonderful subdivision across Ind. 37 from where we lived. He landscaped it, got a bridge built over the creek and put in roads. His brother Don and daughter Amber and her husband Jim built a unique house on the top of a hill toward the back of the addition. Later, Don and his wife Judy would build a custom home just down from Amber and Jim. We were going to join our family members on another lot in the addition with a pond in the sloped backyard.

We were able to sell some of the other lots and were able to pay off a couple of our rentals. God's timing in all of this allowed us to have a regular income without Jerry continuing to work.

My husband built a model of the house, which would have had a walk-out family room or basement area and patio to the pond. He would tinker with it now and then, but finally, we were ready to get started.

We were set to take a trip to Maine with our dear friends Darlene and John. But before we were to leave, several tornados raced through the area, leaving pine trees without their tops, ramming limbs into a couple of the new houses in Jerry's subdivision and tossing much of his carefully planted landscape all over the acreage.

Somehow, it seemed like impending doom. I was at work at the *Reporter-Times* in Martinsville as a news reporter and editor when the storms hit. We hid in the press room, but could see the blackness pass us by hurling birds, signs and debris along as it went. Our roof rattled and we feared for our lives. It devastated many areas and shopping centers around town and took a path down Ind. 37 to the north.

Jerry could see it hit the subdivision and tried to tell me about it as we spoke on our cell phones.

"You won't believe this — oh Amy, oh Amy! It's taking our trees!—" All of a sudden our phones were cut off.

It took me more than an hour to get home, and all the while, I wondered if I still had a house. I realized we were spared, but the subdivision was not.

We went ahead on our trip, putting all the work we had to do over there in the hands of our son and others for a few days.

After 30-some years of marriage, Jerry had become a Christian. I had almost given up hope he would go to church with me, but because of a bout with depression over work and terrible migraine headaches, he went to our doctor, who was already a believer.

He urged my husband to read the Gospel of John in the Bible and wrote it on a prescription paper with some migraine medicine. He still carries that prescription in his wallet.

After Jerry's Promise Keepers experience, his faith became strong and we sat together in the pew. But there was something we didn't know.

God was preparing us both for a struggle we wouldn't be able to handle alone.

> **Psalm 121 (NIV Study Bible)**
>
> I lift up my eyes to the hills, from where does my help come? My help comes from the Lord, maker of Heaven and Earth.
>
> He will not let your foot slip — he who watches over you will not slumber. Indeed, he who watches over Israel will neither slumber nor sleep.
>
> The Lord watches over you, the Lord is your shade at your right hand; the sun will not harm you by day, nor the moon by night.
>
> The Lord will keep you from all harm — he will watch over your life; the Lord will watch over your coming and going both now and forevermore.

A change in plans

I noticed on the trip to Maine that Jerry was tired all the time. Sleep didn't rest him. He would nod off in the car when John was driving even early in the day. He had sores on his arms and legs that looked like bug bites. He had been out in the woods trying to clean up after the tornado, so we thought he had attracted some chiggers.

But they wouldn't heal. Jerry was also breathless after walking a short way. This wasn't like him at all. He was always very physical — an outdoorsman.

When we got home, he went for a physical and continued trying to clean up the mess in Auburn Ridge. A routine blood test showed that he was severely anemic. Our doctor, who knew our histories, was alarmed over this. He sent Jerry to a hematologist.

I was at work when my husband called me, saying it was a kind of leukemia. The doctor was still doing blood work, so we finally got together when I returned home. His face was ashen.

"They got the tests back — it's the worst kind of leukemia," he said with his head in his hands. "It's Acute Lymphocytic Leukemia like young children die of. I'm only 50 years old; my life is just beginning."

We called the pastor of our church and asked him to pray. Instead, Pastor Jim Taylor and his wife Sharon came to our home and comforted us. We all prayed, and Jim reminded Jerry that God was in control. At church that Sunday, all our friends and even people who didn't know us laid hands on Jerry and prayed. His father and Jerry's stepmother Mary Ann joined them.

We were ready to hear the worst.

Not much time to decide

The plan of action for my husband's leukemia was spelled out for us in the oncologist's office at St. Francis Hospital. There were two doctors consulting with each other who worked at St. Francis and IU Medical Center. Dr. Michael Dugan, a bone-marrow transplant specialist and hematologist, had published the protocol for Jerry's treatment, and our main oncologist was Dr. Sharif Khan, also a leukemia researcher.

At once I noticed they were taping everything as we talked.

That's in case things don't work out; we won't be able to claim a lack of communication about Jerry's chances, I thought.

We asked if we could seek another oncologist's opinion.

"You don't have much time," said Dr. Khan. "Jerry has probably had this for a year or more. If treatment isn't begun right away, he only has a few months to survive."

We learned through a bone marrow test that more than 80 percent of the white T-cells used in defending the body from germ invasions were malformed. For all practical purposes, they were useless and crowded out the healthy red blood cells and platelets.

The treatment options were simple. Jerry could have a bone marrow transplant from a relative with healthy T-cells. If a match wasn't found, he was in for a brutal two or three-year regimen of chemotherapy mixed with radiation, Prednisone and blood transfusions.

The risks were explained in detail. The chemo used was capable of damaging small nerve endings and could make my husband deaf, partially blind and permanently numb in his toes and fingers. This type of leukemia often travels up the spine to the brain, so radiation had to be done immediately to prevent that from happening.

But even if everything went according to plan and remission could be achieved, Jerry read on the

Internet that he had only a 30 percent chance of living five years. His age was against him, and the doctors said if he had been in his 60s, he probably would not have been able to survive the treatments at all.

If the cancer returned, Jerry's only chance would be a random bone marrow match and transplant. He could never endure the chemo again.

Doctors said their goal was to bring him into remission.

He could die from a random disease that took hold while his immune system was destroyed in a bone marrow transplant. His kidneys could fail in the midst of a chemo regimen; he could contract a deadly viral pneumonia and become incapable of breathing on his own.

Jerry's brothers were willing to be tested to see if they were a match. We might also find a match in first cousins. Sadly, Don and Gary matched each other, but they didn't match Jerry.

We knew what we were in for and realized our dream of building a new home was out of the question. Luckily, I had been on my company's insurance for two years or we would have faced medical bankruptcy. As it was we had to revisit our will, make decisions about end-of-life options and plans for our sons' inheritance.

Then there was Dr. Khan. The imposing Pakistani native was probably 6 feet, 4 inches tall with black hair and tender dark eyes. He always wore a smile and encouraged us at every turn.

I was torn about this and I admit it now. Because of 9/11, he represented a race of people we were supposed to hate. Yet, I was trusting this kind doctor with my husband's life.

Jerry asked Dr. Khan if he believed a person could be cured by prayer and the laying on of hands.

He was quiet for a moment. I knew he might be a Muslim and thought he would brush off our Christian point of view.

Instead he smiled and said, "Yes, I have heard of this happening. But can I not be considered as part of God's plan for healing?"

We both nodded, "Yes." And from then on we were all in the fight together.

We were almost without hope, but a test was done on Jerry that changed our perspective. Dr. Khan reported that he wasn't a carrier of the Philadelphia chromosome. We had never heard of this, but in Dr. Khan's research, people who carried this chromosome usually had their cancers — especially blood cancers — return after treatment.

"This is a good day, a very good day," He said. We hadn't had one of those in awhile.

John 14:9 Jesus answers his disciple Philip's question on his identity.

> Jesus answered, 'Don't you know me, Philip, even after I have been with you such a long time? Anyone who has seen me has seen the Father. How can you say, Show us the Father. Don't you believe that I am in the Father, and that the Father is in me? The words I say to you are not just my own. Rather it is the Father, living in me, who is doing his work.'

Our support network

In my long relationship with the Lord, I have learned that for every difficult journey, He provides people and entities of support. I shared our upcoming trial with my co-workers. They not only comforted me, they prayed with me and for us.

My managing editor at the time was the legendary Bette Nunn, who ran the *Reporter-Times* when I was first employed there. I had started at the *Mooresville-Decatur Times* and switched to the

Martinsville office to head up our version of the *Hoosier Times* Sunday product.

Our publisher was Jim Kroemer, who told me the staff would support me however I needed them to.

I had formed a prayer alliance with a co-worker at the Mooresville paper, Karen Keeton. After nearly 18 years as prayer partners, we still meet almost every week for lunch or to pray. We've won many battles with our prayers.

We prayed for all kinds of things; our children, husbands, work relationships and people at our churches.

We decided to keep at it even though I was traveling to Martinsville. Once a week we would meet in our cars at her church, Mt. Gilead, and pray before we went to work. At the same time we became members of a small group with our pastor and his wife. These connections would help Jerry and I keep our sanity for the next three years.

My husband developed a closer relationship to his father, who lived with his wife not far from us. The two would eat together and Willard would sometimes go with him to chemotherapy. He had lost two sons already — one from the AIDS virus and the other from a tragic suicide. He asked God to spare him his other sons. And God was faithful.

Jerry entered remission almost right away and never really fell out of it, although he nearly lost his life two times due to the treatments.

His kidneys began to fail, and doctors were frantic trying to find a drug that would turn it around. A nurse was searching clinical trials with Dr. Khan, and they found one that had proven successful in restoring kidney function to patients receiving chemotherapy.

I wasn't sure if our insurance would pay for it, but doctors assured us it had been approved by the Federal Drug Administration and was being used on the East Coast. It was flown to Indianapolis in less than two days. As soon as Jerry began receiving it, his condition improved. We had dodged a bullet.

I spent many nights in a recliner visiting Jerry. I usually didn't stay until morning because I had to keep working. One day, while he was on the sixth floor of St. Francis Hospital in Beech Grove taking a treatment, one of the nurses called me.

"Mr. Hillenburg is having a hard time breathing. He has a viral pneumonia that's common to leukemia patients. We are putting him on oxygen to help him breathe easier. We thought we should call you. We're not sure yet how serious this is," she said.

I had been pushing a deadline on the Sunday paper and trying to finish a story for the *Reporter*. It was too much. I put my head in my hands and the tears came. I knew I had to go to my husband.

Bette heard me crying in the next office and came to put her arms around me. "Do you have to leave?" she asked.

"Yes, they don't know how bad it is yet, and I don't know how long I will have to be with Jerry," I sobbed. "I'm about out of vacation days."

Without skipping a beat, Bette said, "Well, I'm not. I'm going to ask the company to allow you to have a week of my time off."

This wasn't an approved corporate practice. But our controller got the publisher's OK on the switch.

My son Chris and his girlfriend Paula gathered with us, and our son Clay came home as well. Some friends of ours and Jerry's brother Don and sister-in-law Judy, his dad and Mary Ann prayed by his bedside as he struggled with the unknown virus.

I saw the looks on their faces— it told me they thought this might be the last time they saw my husband alive. Later, when everyone was gone, one of the doctors called me outside the room.

"If the medication doesn't work, we will need to take a piece of Jerry's lung to determine what kind of viral pneumonia we are dealing with," the doctor said. "He will probably have to go on a ventilator until we can find the right drugs to fight this."

I slept fitfully in a recliner by Jerry most of the night. He had always said he never wanted to be put on a breathing machine. What was I to do? I continued to pray and ask God to intervene.

All of a sudden, about 2 a.m. the next morning, Jerry flung his legs over the bed. I had noticed his respiration was improving from the monitor. He had been using a bed pan because he was too weak to get up.

"I have to go to the bathroom, he said simply, and began to pull himself up and walked a little unsteadily to the one in the room. I jumped up to help him walk, but he waived me aside. From then on, he continued to recover. Never again would he face death.

Oddly, he was at peace with dying and said, "I thought to myself that if I die, I will see God and be in paradise. And if I live, I will be here with my family — either way — I win," Jerry said about that scary time.

John 14:1-4
Do not let your hearts be troubled. Trust in God, trust also in me. In my Father's house are many rooms; if it were not so, I would have told you. I am going there to prepare a place for you. And if I go and prepare a place for you, I will come back and take you to be with me that you also may be where I am. You know the way to the place where I am going.

CHAPTER 2

A Nun with a Purpose

Since Jerry was in St. Francis Hospital, there were often nuns who stopped by to speak with families if they had designated "Christian" on their registration and admission documents. One sister we could never forget came into my husband's room on the sixth floor. We told her about his religious experience and that he was again attending church.

Jerry was deeply involved, even from his hospital bed, in setting our affairs in order, paying bills and making sure our mortgage and insurance documents were stable for the duration. He was preparing our life in case I would be left a widow. He had boxes of papers stacked in the hospital room.

The nun returned one day and saw what Jerry had been working on. She sat down beside his bed and smiled at both of us.

"You've been worrying about a lot of things," she nodded her head toward the boxes. "But all this will be waiting for you when you get better. Right now, you are in a unique position to use your faith."

We both waited for her to say more, but she measured her words.

"You have a captive audience here. Every day there are nurses and doctors with problems and heartaches only they know about, and they don't believe there's a God who exists to help them — who loves them," she said.

You can tell them about your experience and how it changed you. And you can talk about God every time one of them comes to offer care, a treatment or a meal; even those who clean your room. They have to do their jobs, they can't just walk away."

The sister asked Jerry if he had ever written down his testimony to share with other people.

"I wrote one in 1997 after I came to Christ," Jerry said. "I haven't looked at it for awhile to check it for spelling, but I've written a prayer to go with it since I got diagnosed."

The nun knew that I worked for a local newspaper.

"Your wife can help you with that," she said as she left the room. She poked her head back in the room for one more comment. "Use your time here wisely."

Jerry and I looked at each other. What the nun had said was so profound we had no words to discuss it.

The next day, although my husband was feeling a little weak and nauseous from the chemotherapy, he had me bring him his testimony and prayer to fine-tune it and make copies.

We tried to think of people and relatives we knew who weren't involved in church or who were disillusioned by religious groups. When we felt the testimony and prayer were just right, we made more than 20 copies of them.

Jerry mailed them out or personally gave them to hospital staff or friends who were down or had an obstacle they were facing.

There were many positive reactions to Jerry's testimony, but in only a few cases did we know that an impact had been made. Some people called him and some sent him an email or a letter. We weren't privileged to find out all the results of my husband's attempt to reach out.

The sister told us that God would use Jerry's testimony in a mighty way, and we didn't need to know the intricate details of his plans.

We were able to share this story in our small groups, in Sunday school classes and to parents and families who brought their children to play Upward Basketball.

> **Romans 12:9-13**
> Love must be sincere. Hate what is evil, cling to what is good. Be devoted to one another in brotherly love. Honor one another above yourselves. Never be lacking in zeal, but keep your spiritual fervor, serving the Lord. Be joyful in hope, patient in affliction, faithful in prayer. Share with God's people who are in need. Practice hospitality.

Then there was Fred

When Jerry ran his business, he usually kept a crew of three or four guys. "Fred" was one of them. He had a rather rough personality, shaggy brown hair and would sometimes launch into a few choice cuss words. He liked to have a good time, and he had a kind heart.

More than anything, Fred loved a good joke. He was very talented in trimming out houses, careful and reliable.

Fred was married more than once and took on the responsibility of a father. I never knew if he believed in God — if he did, he didn't share that information. He had left our business a few years back, and we lost track of him.

As Jerry began his intensive chemotherapy, one day ran into the other. I worked during the day and tried to be with him at night. Nurses came in with masks, gowns and double gloves to give him the I-V chemo. He had a three-pronged intravenous hookup in his aorta for the drugs, fluids and anti-nausea medicine he needed.

"Something is wrong with this picture," Jerry laughed one day at the nurses. "You're putting this stuff in my veins, but you guys can't touch it."

They would smile and tell him to imagine the drugs were clearing out all the bad white cells. They said thinking positive was the way to beat cancer.

My husband's hair had already started to thin out on top. But after one strong chemo, he raised his head from the pillow to see the stark-white pillowcase covered in black hair. I always loved his shiny black hair. His family was part Cherokee, and it was one of the things that attracted me to him.

As Jerry looked back on what he had "left behind," the tears came down his cheeks. I had never seen him cry before, and he quickly wiped his face. I put my hand on his shoulder and kissed him.

"I'll go down to the nurses' station and get you a Coke. Try to rest now and don't worry, they say it usually grows back," I said, trying to comfort him.

Both of us were low that day.

As I walked down the quiet hall (it was a weekend at the hospital), I noticed two men striding toward me in suits and ties and Bibles in their hands. Immediately, I noticed the bright blue eyes and crooked smile of one of the prayer partners. It was Fred. His hair was cropped neatly, and he had slimmed down quite a bit.

"What are you doing here, Fred?" I asked, noticing the well-worn Good Book he clutched.

"Why are you on this floor?" he returned my question. "Is it one of the boys?"

Fred had always been very fond of our two sons who worked part-time for the business in the summers.

"No, it's Jerry, and it isn't good, Fred. He has an acute form of leukemia, and we're starting the radiation and chemotherapy," I said.

I tried to sound strong, but Fred and the other man could tell I had been crying. They shared that they came often to the hospital to pray with patients, visiting with them and telling others about God's love.

They "just happened" to be on the sixth floor that day. Fred looked at me in disbelief.

Right away, there in the hall, the two men laid their hands on my head and prayed out loud for Jerry and I. The words filled me with a strength I had been lacking — the strength to continue.

The two of them went into Jerry's room, and I could hear them laughing, praying together and recalling old times.

Fred told of his conversion to Christianity and how he had straightened out many things in his life. My husband began to smile again and kept saying over and over, "Fred in a coat and tie holding a Bible — I don't believe it, I don't believe it."

I treasured that spontaneous gift from the Lord. It was just what we needed; an old friend to give us a new perspective on how God can change lives in an instant. I will never forget it.

> **2 Corinthians 4:6-9**
> For God, who said, 'Let the light shine out of the darkness,' made his light shine in our hearts to give us the light of knowledge of the glory of God in the face of Christ. But we have this treasure in jars of clay to show that this all-surpassing power is from God and not from us. We are hard-pressed on every side, but not crushed; perplexed, but not in despair; persecuted, but not abandoned; struck down, but not destroyed.

And God lit the way

It had not been a good day for me — or my husband. Jerry's kidneys were acting up again, and medications the hospital had tried weren't working. He had received an especially aggressive chemo, which was known to cause trouble in the bladder and kidneys. It had kept him in remission, though.

I was weary sitting in the recliner by my husband's bed and waiting for doctors to come and go and tell us what was going on. Jerry seemed to be getting weaker. His skin was a pale yellow color, and he had a weird coating on his tongue. I had to go home and get some sleep.

I took the following day off, and a dear church friend Marti called to ask how things were going. She and her husband Gene lived in Mooresville, just northeast of our home in Waverly.

As we were talking, the stress of the day came to a head, and I dissolved into tears. Gene was an associate pastor at our church, and they both offered to pray for me. Then Marti asked if I wanted to come spend the night at their home — she didn't want me to be alone in my house.

I agreed. It would be nice to have some company. The weather was stormy, and an intense rainstorm was just coming to an end as I pulled my car out of the hospital garage.

I had only been on the highway for about 15 minutes when the sky began to clear and a brilliant, full rainbow appeared in front of me. It crossed the entire highway. I had seen partial rainbows before, but never one like this.

A few drivers actually pulled over to look at it, taking their life in their hands as other vehicles sped past them.

A warm feeling of peace enveloped me as I drove and gazed at the rainbow. I felt it was the Lord telling me that no matter what problems my husband was facing, He was in control of the universe. We had nothing to fear — not in this world or the next. For the first time in a week, I experienced a sound sleep at Marti and Gene's house. They fixed me breakfast, prayed with me and watched as I drove away.

At the hospital, one of the nurses told me Jerry had tried to get out of the leukemia ward via the elevator. He simply unplugged his wires and was still in his hospital gown when nurses spotted him.

"That looks like Mr. Hillenburg That *is* Mr. Hillenburg!" one of them yelled. He told them he was ready to go home, but they were able to coax him back to his room. The next day he was feeling better but was embarrassed over his attempted elevator escape. He felt he was causing everyone trouble with his night terrors.

"I'm going to beat this, Amy. You'll see," Jerry said, grabbing my hand. It was another long night, but by morning, his kidneys were back to normal. However, my husband's body chemistry had gone awry, and he began to have the hiccups. They were so violent they shook the bed. Several times I had to leave the room — I couldn't stand to see him suffering.

Doctors had cures for cancer, but there was almost nothing they could do for hiccups except to sedate Jerry. He even hiccupped in his sleep. The onslaught lasted three days. By drinking plenty of water and eating a certain diet, the hiccups subsided. His chest muscles were sore, and he laughed saying now I shouldn't mind his snoring. He was right, never would I mind his snoring again.

> **Genesis 9:13-15**
> I have set my rainbow in the clouds, and it will be a sign of the covenant between me and the earth. Whenever I bring clouds over the earth and the rainbow appears in the clouds, I will remember my covenant between me and you and all living creatures of every kind. Never again will the waters become a flood to destroy all life.

Patient reinforcement

Jerry had been struggling with one physical setback after another. Our reserves were low. God knew we needed help to go the extra mile, and one day a man about my husband's age appeared at the door of his room. I can't recall his name, but he looked fit and was tan from a recent trip to Florida.

He introduced himself and began telling Jerry that several years ago, he was diagnosed with the same leukemia. We could hardly believe it.

Like Jerry, he had a long-standing marriage and was a father of grown children.

"You're in good hands," the man told us. "Your doctors are the best in the field. They changed my diet and I started an exercise regimen. There were a couple of times when I almost died. But I've been clear of leukemia now for five years."

He shook Jerry's hand, and it was as if my husband got an infusion of strength and health from this man's sturdy grip.

"I know you're not feeling too good right now, but you will get better. Someday you can call me up and we'll go fishing," he smiled.

Jerry didn't fish, but it was a wonderful dream just the same.

"And your doctor is right — stay off the Internet. Remember that even if 70 percent of leukemia patients don't make it five years, 30 percent go on to have pretty normal lives. I'm one of them."

Because he came to visit, Jerry and I were good for another few months. It wasn't until a year or so later that we learned the man had died. We went to the showing, and his wife was in shock.

"He was doing so well," she said to us. "He got a lung infection and kept putting off going to the doctor. When he did, they put him in the hospital, and in three days he was dead." A tear streamed down her cheek.

"I'm glad to see you so well, Jerry. Just remember if you get sick, don't wait — go to the doctor."

That advice held us in good stead three years later when my husband got pneumonia. He ended up in the emergency room but was able to recover because of that brave woman's words.

> **2 Corinthians 1:3-5**
> Praise be to the God and Father of the Lord Jesus Christ, the Father of compassion and the God of all comfort; who comforts us in all our troubles, so that we can comfort those in any trouble with the comfort we ourselves have received from God. For just as the sufferings of Christ flow over into our lives, so also through Christ our comfort overflows.

CHAPTER 3

My Story

How I came to know Christ

Jerry Hillenburg, 1997

When I was young, my family attended a church that required us to live by some rather odd rules. Rules like: no Boy Scouts allowed, no TVs, no dancing and no movies. If you had friends outside the church, shame on you.

These rules were designed to protect us from what the church leaders called the "sinful world." Well, as soon as we were old enough, my brothers and I left that church, fast. If this was how God wanted us to worship, then forget it. Now I understand that such rules are not made by God, but by man.

When I reached middle age, I visited my doctor because of health problems. All the tests came back negative so the doctor quizzed me about my spiritual life. He explained that a human being is like a three-legged stool. One leg is the physical body, the second our mental being and the third leg is our spiritual being. If one of these legs is missing or weak, the stool can't function properly.

The next Sunday, I attended church for the first time in 30 years. The following week, I again visited my doctor and proudly told him of my church visit. He said, "That's great, but taking up pew space will not get your spiritual life in order, you have to invite Christ to come into your life through prayer." He gave me a prescription paper, and on it he had wrote, "Gospel of John." He said, "Read this chapter of the Bible and then you will better understand how to have a relationship with Christ."

About a year later, I woke up in the middle of the night because of a deep emptiness inside me. I felt I had no reason to continue life, and for the first time in my adult life, I cried. That night I decided to go to an upcoming Christian men's conference and maybe there I could find a cure for this terrible emptiness.

At the meeting, a member of the group I was with prayed with me, and I invited Jesus Christ into my life. On the way home I pulled off to the side of the road, and for the second time in my adult life, I cried. But this time it was for the joy of knowing Christ!

It took me 45 years to understand I was made with a God-shaped hole in my heart. I tried to fill that hole with other things, but now I know only God will fit. I have even more health problems now and my life isn't perfect. But the emptiness I felt in the past is gone because I know Jesus Christ is always there for me. As an added benefit I have the gift of eternal life!

— Jerry Hillenburg, 1997

My diagnosis was Acute Leukemia; my prayer is...

Dear God, I feel like a little shepherd boy with a slingshot facing a giant named Cancer. It is more than I can handle, but it is not more than You can handle. The shepherd's battle cry was not "I know I can't, I know I can't" but it was "I know God can, I know God can." Like the shepherd boy, I am going to let You fight the giant.

I pray desperately for a cure, but I do not know if You will cure me. I do know You are going to work in my life; the future is determined by Your perfect way. My focus is on You, God, not the giant. I fear nothing, and I am excited about my future! In Jesus Christ's name, Amen.

CHAPTER 4

A Dog from My Mother

In 1987, I lost my beloved mother to a rare autoimmune disease called Scleroderma. She fought it for almost 11 years, but the runaway collagen in her body wrapped itself around her lungs. She died on the respirator after about four months in and out of the hospital — and lost a leg in the process.

My dad followed her soon after in 1989, succumbing to lung cancer after more than 60 years of heavy smoking. It felt at the time like a hole had been ripped out of my soul. I was close to both my parents and talked to them every week; if not every day.

When Jerry got sick and at times of crisis, I could actually feel their presence. Both were Christians, and I knew that heaven was their home. I don't know how those who've passed into eternity see or are aware of what goes on down here. But the bonds that bind family are nearly unbreakable.

My mother loved dogs and took in every stray cat or mutt that climbed up our front porch.

My dad did not always agree with the animal personalities that shared our home. Since none of them were pure-bred, they each had their idiosyncrasies. One pretty dog that we called "Heidi" was terribly shy and only came to the living room if it was just us sitting around. If a stranger came into our midst, she escaped to a braided rug where she stayed until he, she or they left.

Another male cat used to leave for two or three days in a row and come back with a chewed up ear, blood on his paws or a missing tooth. My mother constantly worked with animal character flaws until the dogs and cats in our home began to show their love for us. It was amazing to see the transformation.

When Jerry got out of the hospital, he drove himself to chemotherapy treatments, sometimes with his dad along. But with me still working he was lonely during the day. Our cat "Peanut Butter" laid down one afternoon under a chair and died after 21 years. We were all heartbroken. It was time to get another animal.

Jerry was told by his doctors that bacteria from litter boxes could bring infection to him, and with his weakened immune system, a rare pneumonia or flu could take his life. So we discussed a dog.

"I'd like to get a pure-bred dog — I know we'll have to pay for it, but a small little fluffy dog would be great. I could take it with me wherever I go and hold it in my lap after chemo," Jerry said.

My husband researches everything he intends to buy and created a short list of dogs that pleased him and also did not shed. I was agreeable to the plan, and we began to look up breeders in the area.

At the same time, a friend of mine stopped by at the *Reporter-Times* office in Martinsville. She asked to see me, so I went up front. Susan was excited.

"Amy, I heard you wanted to get a dog for Jerry. I've got the perfect one for you at the Humane Society shelter. She's beautiful, and she's been so abused," Susan said. "Her owner hasn't been feeding her, so she's hungry and cold — then she came in heat. All the neighborhood dogs were after her. A man who lived near her owner couldn't stand to see her suffering, so he put her in the back of his truck and took her to the shelter."

"What kind of dog is she?" I asked, hoping against hope the dog was pure-bred.

"No, she's a mix, but she looks like the dog on the Purina Dog Chow bags," my friend said. "Just go and see her; if you do, you'll take her home."

My whole animal history was based on strays, shelter dogs and mutts. Reluctantly I went over to the shelter. I didn't tell Jerry right away. I knew what he wanted.

Babe had her face in the corner of the pen with her tail tucked under her legs. Two big dogs were barking in the pens next to her and scaring her to death. She was a wavy-haired white dog with some yellowish streaks in her fur. She had a little beard, soft fluffy ears and furry feet.

"We've been calling her 'Baby,' the volunteer worker said. "She's real afraid and she's been chased by other dogs a lot. I will get her for you."

"Baby" was very pretty and a smaller mid-size dog. I reached out for her and she immediately came into my arms. She was shivering and so fearful.

"How old is she?" I asked the attendant.

"The vet thinks she's not much more than a year old because her teeth are still pretty clean. We don't know if she's potty trained, but she's used to going outside. We take her out on a leash," he said.

I knew instinctively that God had sent this dog to us. Jerry needed healing and "Baby" needed love and company. It was a perfect pairing. I just needed to convince him to take a shelter dog. She would have to be spayed first and receive her shots.

This was the kind of dog my mother would have taken home. Mom's friends always called her by Dad's pet name for her, "Babe." I decided that if we got this dog, that would be her name.

I told Jerry at supper that night about this lovely female dog that needed a home.

"I thought we agreed on a pure-bred," Jerry said. "And I wanted more of a lap dog. I don't know. She'll probably be afraid of everything and then what will we do with her?"

"Do me a favor; just go to the shelter to see her one time. If you still want to go the other route, we will," I said.

Okay, okay, I will go over there," my husband said reluctantly.

He was gone a long time, and I couldn't figure out what was happening. Suddenly I heard the sound of his van in the driveway. It was still light outside and to my surprise, "Babe" was sitting beside Jerry in the passenger seat. It was almost as if the spot had been made for her.

Babe served my husband and me as our faithful companion for almost 12 years before she died from an unknown bowel blockage on our bathroom floor with us by her side.

We cried off and on for weeks, but we hoped since God sent her to us, he would keep her in heaven for when we get there.

> **Luke 12:6, 7**
> Are not two sparrows sold for a penny? Yet, not one of them will fall to the ground apart from the will of your Father. And even the very hairs of your head are all numbered. So don't be afraid; you are worth more than many sparrows.

My other mothers — and brother

Since my mother died when I was only 36 years old, I've been amazed at the number of older

A Dog from My Mother

women God has put in my life. They've been mentors, friends, comforters and advisors.

I will start with my mom's sisters Charlotte and Helen — and my cousin Jean Ann. At the holidays after my mother passed before Thanksgiving, they made sure we all went to Brown County the day after. We shopped, ate and were able to celebrate a little bit, despite the sadness we felt about Mom.

We made that a tradition and journeyed to Nashville, Indiana, for the next three or four years after Thanksgiving. My aunts and cousin called me regularly and loved for me to visit them whenever possible.

Willard and Mary Ann also took special care to ask us to church and to other family events.

My aunts and cousins Donna and Sue on my dad's side also kept in touch with me and tried to have get-togethers every few months. Although Hilda died at age 92, Betty and Miriam are still alive and two very vital women.

My Aunt Helen had never driven a car, so sometimes I would take her to the grocery and out to eat.

She was not in good health and actually leaned over the shopping cart to endure the hour in the store. She refused an automated wheelchair, saying she was going to keep going as long as she could. Helen's two sons lived not too far from her, but she didn't get out very much.

Helen, who has passed away, lived alone as did Charlotte. Both women had lost their husbands and were still in their own homes. Yet they kept going. Jean Ann and her husband Art moved in with Charlotte when she entered her 90s and was no longer able to safely drive a car.

My brother Allen has been my rock. His recent death following open-heart surgery was a shock and devastating loss to me. He and his wife suffered from addiction in their early life, but got sober and resumed their marriage and Christian faith.

I cherished their care of me and that they always listened when I had problems in my own family. Their sobriety was a special gift from God. He knew I would need my brother and sister-in-law in the coming years.

On more than one occasion, I sought the hugs and welcoming arms of my relatives when I just wanted to cry in frustration during Jerry's illness. Although they didn't look just like my mother, her sisters were all I had left of her — and it was enough to get me through.

Other older women entered my life at different times to supply a need for motherly comfort and encouragement. Although I don't have contact with some of them anymore, I treasured their friendship at the time.

God often puts people in our lives for a season and sometimes removes them for one reason or another. We shouldn't grieve over that or feel guilty that the friendships have gone their way. Everyone we meet adds value to our character and helps us mature. Or, they bring out talents we didn't know we had.

As my late editor Bette Nunn used to say, "Not everyone will become your dearest friend and some may not like you at all. Accept that, go on and take as much as you can from every relationship. Give people the benefit of the doubt. If you haven't walked in their shoes, you don't know what they're dealing with."

I've never forgotten that advice.

> **Ruth 1:16**
> But Ruth replied, "Don't urge me to leave you or to turn back from you. Where you go I will go, and where you stay I will stay. Your people will be my people and your God my God."

Ecclesiastes 4:12
Though one may be overpowered, two can defend themselves. But a cord of three strands is not quickly broken.

The greatest gift of all

For almost three years, my husband fought off his acute leukemia with chemo, radiation and steroids — sometimes in combination and sometimes by themselves. His doctors finally released him from treatment.

No one ever says you're cured of blood-related cancer. But they say you are "maintaining remission."

We were glad to accept that description of his new hold on life. He was required to get blood tests two or three times a year for awhile. But for once, he could eat what he wanted like fried mushrooms, do some physical things, be among crowds of people and welcome a newcomer to our family.

My oldest son Chris had been divorced for a couple of years. We were all down about it, but he finally met another woman who seemed to make him happy. After two years of marriage, his wife Paula found she was pregnant.

It was no secret that I had always wanted a little girl. But God had decided to give the girls to my brother Allen. He had two of his own and adopted another.

I felt as if they were my daughters. They stayed overnight at our house, went on outings with me, played girl games and loved the frilly clothes I bought them.

After Jerry recovered, Paula learned she would have a little girl. We were ecstatic. I jumped up and down and screamed when Chris told me the news over the phone.

It was as if God was giving us a reward for all Jerry's suffering. During Paula's labor, it was decided the baby was taking too long to come down the birth canal. Doctors decided to take her Caesarian section. She was born three hours away from Jerry's own birthday, Oct. 27. He had been born on his mother's birthday.

The precious little girl was perfect in every way. Chris came down the hallway dressed in a hospital gown and gloves. We thought he was the doctor. Our youngest son Clay had come home that week, and as Chris pulled the blanket back he said, "She looks just like you, Mom.

Paula and Chris named her Naomi from the Bible. It was kind of unsettling, looking at her little features and noticing they closely resembled my own baby pictures.

Naomi is like me and her father in so many ways. She loves art and music, likes helping others, craves adventure and loves planting flowers and shopping for the latest fashions. From the time she was a baby, Naomi has always smiled and laughed — and she loves kidding Jerry, her "Pawpaw."

Once he teased her about losing all of her front teeth. One Sunday during the ride to church, he called her his "little toothless thing."

Naomi thought for a moment as if trying to find the right reply. Suddenly she patted Jerry's bald head.

"My teeth will grow back, but your hair will never grow back," she giggled.

We are always amazed at her sense of humor and her ability to get along with almost everybody. She is our only grandchild, but God gave us a lovely and perfect one. We can never praise him enough for this greatest gift of all.

James 1:17

Every good and perfect gift is from above, coming down from the Father of heavenly lights, who does not change like shifting shadows."

Matthew 18:10

See that you do not despise one of these little ones. For I tell you that their angels in heaven always see the face of my Father in heaven.

CHAPTER 5

A Hot-Air Celebration

For one year, Jerry had received normal blood tests — no more trace of leukemia. Doctors aren't always great at saying you are cured. They say things like, "We know the cancer is probably hiding somewhere, but our microscopes aren't powerful enough to see it. So, you can go back to once a year physicals with a blood test to check for leukemia."

It meant a freedom my husband and I had not known for almost three years. I wanted a wonderful way to celebrate, and as it happened, the experience fell right into my lap.

My father's sister Aunt Betty was turning 80. She was known in her circle of friends as the "Hat Lady."

She collects hats for all occasions, and to date has 110 in her possession. They are of every color and theme; she matches them to her clothing or the occasion.

Betty had arranged to have a hot-air balloon ride on her birthday with her granddaughter's balloon company. She felt safe with the owners because they often flew government officials and celebrities in their balloons.

She bought tickets for her and her daughter, my cousin Donna. There was one problem with this plan. Donna hated heights and told my aunt she would have to find a stand-in for her balloon ride.

For some reason, Betty and Donna remembered a conversation we had when I said a hot-air balloon ride was something I wanted to experience.

"Amy, you can go with me — I'll give you the ticket as an early birthday present," Betty said.

I felt that I had won the lottery. Jerry wasn't so sure.

"You're kidding; you're not really going to do this are you? You're a grandmother after all. What if something terrible happens?" Jerry said.

I wasn't to be swayed.

Betty and I, Donna and my husband drove to the north side where the balloon was being prepared. We didn't know until the last moment that we would go up that day. Balloons usually went up in the morning and late afternoon, and if there was a wind of at least 10 miles per hour, the trip was postponed.

The balloon company reps sent up regular-sized balloons to check the wind direction. We were going to "float" over to Geist Reservoir. Donna and my husband hovered around us as the balloon was filled with air. This took almost an hour and was done with big electric wind fans.

Once the balloon was up and ready to go, we had to jump quickly into the shoulder-high basket before the helpers let go of the ropes. If you don't move quickly enough, you get left behind. The basket was just large enough for Betty, me, a young boy and the balloonist.

It was a hot day with a light breeze and as dusk set in, we entered the quiet part of the sky far above the traffic, the yards, people, pools and tree lines. There was a mild smell of the gas, but not enough to really bother us.

The balloonist gave each of us miniature parachute men to hoist over the side of the basket. The boy just loved doing it.

Sometimes, we would come face-to-face with some trees. I was sure we were going to hit them. I voiced my fears aloud. The balloonist laughed.

"No, I never hit the trees, we're going up and over them."

And before we knew it, we were soaring over their leafy tops, scattering birds all around. This guy was a master at flying a balloon. We relaxed and enjoyed the ride.

Betty was wearing a jacket, thinking it would be cold in the upper reaches. It was not. She became overheated and a little woozy from the emissions. Suddenly, she sat down in the crowded basket and took off her pink cap.

"I think I'm going to throw up in my hat," she said.

"We don't have to go around the whole Geist Reservoir, we can start heading back right now," the balloonist said.

It was then I heard my phone ring and realized that Jerry and Donna were worried about Betty and had followed our balloon in their vehicles. I didn't know how to tell them my aunt was sick without really upsetting them.

A Hot-Air Celebration

"She's OK, she's been a little woozy but she never did throw up. We're coming down early," I told my cousin.

"Thank God," Donna said. "Where are you going to land?"

The balloonist hovered around a Geist neighborhood with estate-size homes and manicured yards. He was talking on his phone to someone on the ground. He had spotted an empty side-yard of a neighbor that was big enough for us to land on.

Betty was feeling better. Even though she stayed sitting down, she had a little space in the basket through which she could see the wonders of our ride. Although she was disappointed in herself that she hadn't endured it standing up, I told her I was still amazed that she went up in the air at all.

From hearing about other friends' hot air balloon rides, I learned that you could have a rough landing. One of my mother's sisters said her basket had landed partially on its side and she fell onto another passenger who joked that she secretly wanted to get close to him. Betty and I laughed about it, but as the ground came closer and closer, my face began to flush. Sweat beads appeared on my forehead.

Before I let terror overtake me, hands reached out on either side of the basket and pulled us down to a soft landing. And we were upright.

We had a wonderful family dinner where we talked about the high points of the ride. I felt it was like touching heaven. My aunt despaired that she had failed the endeavor. But Betty was vindicated a couple of years later when she rode a zip line my husband built in our yard. I might add, she did it twice, just so her picture could be taken.

Isaiah 40:31
But those who hope in the Lord will renew their strength. They will soar on wings like eagles; they will run and not grow weary, they will walk and not be faint.

Paying it forward

Jerry and I had two dear friends we had come to know at our church. Their names were unusual, Ivan and Vadyes. Both had been married before, and Ivan had grown children from his first marriage. The two of them had one son of their own. They were wonderful caring people and taught in the kids' Sunday school.

A Hot-Air Celebration

We all liked to water ski, and Ivan had a speedboat. After moving a couple of times, he and Vadyes decided to buy a home on a lake. We visited them often for suppers, cards, pool or just to talk.

Our friends always took us on a pontoon boat ride, and one summer we took a trip to Kentucky Lake together on a houseboat. We kept Ivan's speedboat tied up in case we wanted some water adventures.

Ivan loved cars and had his own vehicle repair business. He collected classic cars, painting them and refurbishing them.

We had not heard from Ivan and Vadyes for a while since they began attending another church closer to their home.

One night, we got a call from Vadyes. She said Ivan had been diagnosed with advanced prostate cancer and also had a spot on his spine. We were devastated.

Jerry had recovered well from his leukemia and was healthy, despite having to take afternoon naps to get energy for the evening.

He also had lost most of the hearing in one of his ears. He had to have cataracts removed from his eyes, but these were only pesky inconveniences. We just dealt with them.

Our friends from church suggested we call the couple and pray with and lay hands on Ivan. So quickly, God provided a way for us to pay back what we had received from Him — a new lease on life.

Gladly, we agreed to invite them over for a meal, and members of our Bible study turned out to do what Christians do; pray and trust the Lord.

Ivan and Vadyes were excited that this might turn the course of his cancer treatment journey.

We all laid our hands on his back and prayed for his healing. It was *déjà vu*, for us as we remembered them doing this for Jerry. I know that sometimes healing does not always come, even with prayer. We have lost some young church members to cancer, accidents and other diseases. My friend Marti also died recently from pulmonary fibrosis.

But Vadyes had quite a while to work before she could retire. Ivan's cancer could break them financially. Part of our prayer was for him to have added years with his wife and family.

That was almost eight years ago, and Ivan is still outliving his diagnosis. He, like Jerry, has had to endure some debilitating drugs — especially female hormones.

"I don't know what's wrong with me," Ivan said during one of our visits. "I wake up in the middle of the night in sweats. Sometimes I feel faint, and other days I get upset over the littlest thing. I even teared up over a movie."

Vadyes and I looked at each other and laughed. We knew those symptoms very well. They marked the times we took birth control pills and also when we were about to go into menopause.

"We know just how you feel, Ivan," I said with a wink. We all joked around about it.

There have been some recurrences of his cancer, and he's had a brain scan to watch a troublesome area. But Ivan has remained strong and even bought a building in Martinsville where he and friends could play games, watch TV and listen to music.

In the back, he set up a shop where he could restore classic cars. The project has kept him going and motivated him to sell his business and spend his time in more fulfilling ways.

> **James 5:14 ESV**
>
> Is anyone among you sick? Let him call for the elders of the church and let them pray over him, anointing him with oil in the name of the Lord.

James 5:16 ESV
Therefore, confess your sins to one another and pray for one another, that you may be healed. The prayer of a righteous person has great power as it is working.

God was still working

When Jerry was released from his room in isolation (double windows and visitors in gowns and masks), we prayed over the bed, the windows and all the monitors and furnishings. We asked God to give special healing to all who occupied that room.

A few years after Jerry finished his chemotherapy, we decided to pay a visit to the sixth floor of St. Francis just to thank the nurses who had cared for my husband there. Not all of the same ones were on duty, but there were a couple of them who recognized Jerry and were so happy to see him enjoying good health.

"You know, every patient that we put in that room goes into remission," one of the nurses said.

Jerry and I looked at each other and smiled. It was God still at work on that leukemia ward. We shared the secret of the room's power. The nurses could hardly find the words to react. But one patted my husband's shoulder and said, "Come back again sometime. There are a lot of patients who would be glad to see a survivor."

Jerry and I don't know how much more time we will have together, but we have pledged to spend that time encouraging others in the fight for their health. I thank God for the extra years we've been given. Both of us have learned to lean on the Lord's strength. It is ever-present and everlasting.

> **Psalm 33:4-9**
>
> For the word of the Lord is right and true; he is faithful in all he does. The Lord loves righteousness and justice; the earth is full of his unfailing love.
>
> By the word of the Lord were the heavens made, their starry host in the breath of his mouth. He gathers the waters of the sea into jars; he puts the deep into storehouses.
>
> Let all the earth fear the Lord; let all the people of the world revere him. For he spoke, and it came to be; he commanded, and it stood firm.

About the Author

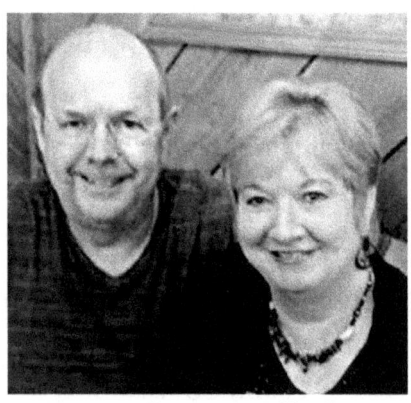

Amy and Jerry Hillenburg

Amy Hillenburg is retired after working 22 years for the *Mooresville-Decatur Times* and *Reporter-Times* in Martinsville as a news reporter, news editor and columnist. She has won awards for her writing from the Hoosier State Press Association and was chosen as the Networking Business Woman of the Year by the NBW organization in Mooresville. She has also written poetry and has published two children's books.

Amy has been married 44 years to Jerry Hillenburg, a former trim carpenter and cabinet specialist. They have two sons, Chris and Clay Hillenburg, and one granddaughter, Naomi Hillenburg. She and Jerry attend Grace Missionary Church in Mooresville. Her hobbies include traveling, reading, writing, gardening, biking, walking and gatherings with friends. Jerry is a 14-year survivor of Acute Lymphocytic Leukemia.

www.ingramcontent.com/pod-product-compliance
Lightning Source LLC
Chambersburg PA
CBHW071123030426
42336CB00013BA/2186